The Plant-Based Diet Cookbook

The Complete Plant-Based CookBook with Delicious Recipes and a Fast 3-Weeks Meal Plan Program to Burn Fat

Vegetarian Academy

© Copyright 2021 by Vegetarian Academy - All rights reserved.

The following Book is reproduced below with the goal of providing information that is as accurate and reliable as possible. Regardless, purchasing this Book can be seen as consent to the fact that both the publisher and the author of this book are in no way experts on the topics discussed within and that any recommendations or suggestions that are made herein are for entertainment purposes only. Professionals should be consulted as needed prior to undertaking any of the action endorsed herein.

This declaration is deemed fair and valid by both the American Bar Association and the Committee of Publishers Association and is legally binding throughout the United States.

Furthermore, the transmission, duplication, or reproduction of any of the following work including specific information will be considered an illegal act irrespective of if it is done electronically or in print. This extends to creating a secondary or tertiary copy of the work or a recorded copy and is only allowed with the express written consent from the Publisher. All additional right reserved.

The information in the following pages is broadly considered a truthful and accurate account of facts and as such, any inattention, use, or misuse of the information in question by the reader will render any resulting actions solely under their purview. There are no scenarios in which the publisher or the original author of this work can be in any fashion deemed liable for any hardship or damages that may befall them after undertaking information described herein.

Additionally, the information in the following pages is intended only for informational purposes and should thus be thought of as universal. As befitting its nature, it is presented without assurance regarding its prolonged validity or interim quality. Trademarks that are mentioned are done without written consent and can in no way be considered an endorsement from the trademark holder.

Tables of Contents

21 DAYS MEAL PLAN 6

THE PLANT BASED BREAKFAST 9

- KETO PORRIDGE 9
- EASY CHIA SEED PUDDING 11
- CINNAMON NOATMEAL 13
- DELICIOUS VEGAN ZOODLES 15
- AVOCADO TOFU SCRAMBLE 17
- CHIA RASPBERRY PUDDING SHOTS 19
- HEALTHY CHIA-ALMOND PUDDING 21
- DELICIOUS TOFU FRIES 22
- FRESH BERRIES WITH CREAM 24
- ALMOND HEMP HEART PORRIDGE 26

THE PLANT BASED LUNCH 28

- AVOCADO & RADISH SALAD 28
- BAKED OKRA & TOMATO 30
- WATERCRESS & BLOOD ORANGE SALAD 32
- LENTIL POTATO SALAD 34
- EDAMAME SALAD 36
- CAULIFLOWER & APPLE SALAD 38
- OLIVE & FENNEL SALAD 40
- RED PEPPER & BROCCOLI SALAD 42
- ZUCCHINI & LEMON SALAD 44
- MEDITERRANEAN WRAP 45
- QUINOA WITH NECTARINE SLAW 47
- SUMMER CHICKPEA SALAD 49
- CORN & BLACK BEAN SALAD 51
- PARSLEY SALAD 53
- RED LENTIL SOUP 55

DINNER RECIPES 57

- TOFU & ASPARAGUS STIR FRY 57
- CAULIFLOWER STEAKS 60
- TOFU POKE 62
- RATATOUILLE 64
- TOMATO GAZPACHO 67
- SIMPLE CHILI 69

THE PLANT-BASED DIET COOKBOOK

- Cauliflower Rice Tabbouleh 71
- Dijon Maple Burgers 73
- Sushi Bowl 75
- Pesto & Tomato Quinoa 77
- Sesame Bok Choy 79
- Stuffed Bell Pepper 81
- Cabbage & Beet Stew 82
- Black Bean Burgers 84
- Grilled Eggplant Steaks 86
- Vegetable Stir Fry 88
- Fried Pineapple Rice 90

SOUP SALADS AND SIDES 92

- Cauliflower Coconut Rice 92
- Fried Okra 94
- Asparagus Mash 96
- Baked Asparagus 98
- Spinach with Coconut Milk 99
- Delicious Cabbage Steaks 100
- Garlic Zucchini Squash 102
- Tomato Avocado Cucumber Salad 104
- Cabbage Coconut Salad 106
- Asian Cucumber Salad 108

21 Days Meal Plan

The plant-based diet is a style of eating that focuses entirely on food from plants. Foods in this category include fruits, nuts, seeds grains, legumes, vegetables, oils, and beans.

The plant-based diet is different from a vegan or vegetarian plan because a plant-based diet doesn't forbid eating animal products; it allows you to choose a more proportionate amount of plant-sourced food in your diet. People understand and use the phrase plant-based diet in a variety of ways; a lot of people take the name literally. For most of those people, the plant-based diet is like a vegan diet where no animal products are involved. But the truth is that the person who is following a plant-based diet can consume chicken, meat, or fish occasionally. The main focus is on the whole and healthy food items rather than the processed items.

Enjoy your meal!
Here's your weekly meal plan.

THE PLANT-BASED DIET COOKBOOK

Days	Breakfast	Lunch	Dinner
1.	Keto Porridge	Avocado & Radish Salad	Tofu & Asparagus Stir Fry
2.	Easy Chia Seed Pudding	Baked Okra & Tomato	Curry Mushroom Pie
3.	Cinnamon Noatmeal	Watercress & Blood Orange Salad	Tofu Poke
4.	Vegan Zuddles	Lentil Potato Salad	Ratattoulle
5.	Avocado Tofu Scramble	Eddame Salad	Tomato Gazpacho
6.	Chia Rasberry Pudding Shots	Cauliflower & Apple Salad	Simple Chili
7.	Healthy Chia-Almond Pudding	Olive & Fennel Salad	Cavuliflowrer RiseTabbouleh
8.	Tofu Fries	Red Pepper & Broccolio Salad	Doun Maple Burgers
9.	Fresh Berries with Cream	Zucchini & Lemon Salad	Sushi Bowl
10.	Almond Hemp Heart Porridge	Mediterranean Wrap	Pesto & Tomato Quinoa
11.	Keto Porridge	Quinoa with Nectarin Slaw	Sesame Bok Choy
12.	Easy Chia Seed Pudding	Summer Chickpea Salad	Stuffed Beel Pepper
13.	Cinnamon Noatmeal	Corn & Black Bean Salad	Cabbage & Beet Stew
14.	Vegan Zuddles	Parsley Salad	Black-Bean Burgers
15.	Avocado Tofu Scramble	REd Lentil Soup	Grilled eggplant sticks

THE PLANT-BASED DIET COOKBOOK

16.	Chia Rasberry Pudding Shots	Avocado & Radish Salad	Vegetable Stir Fry
17.	Healthy Chia-Almond Pudding	Baked Okra & Tomato	Fried Pineapple Rice
18.	Tofu Fries	Cauliflower & Apple Salad	Tofu Poke
19.	Fresh Berries with Cream	Olive & Fennel Salad	Ratattoulle
20.	Almond Hemp Heart Porridge	Red Pepper & Broccolio Salad	Tomato Gazpacho
21.	Cinnamon Noatmeal	Mediterranean Wrap	Stuffed Beel Pepper

The Plant Based Breakfast

Keto Porridge

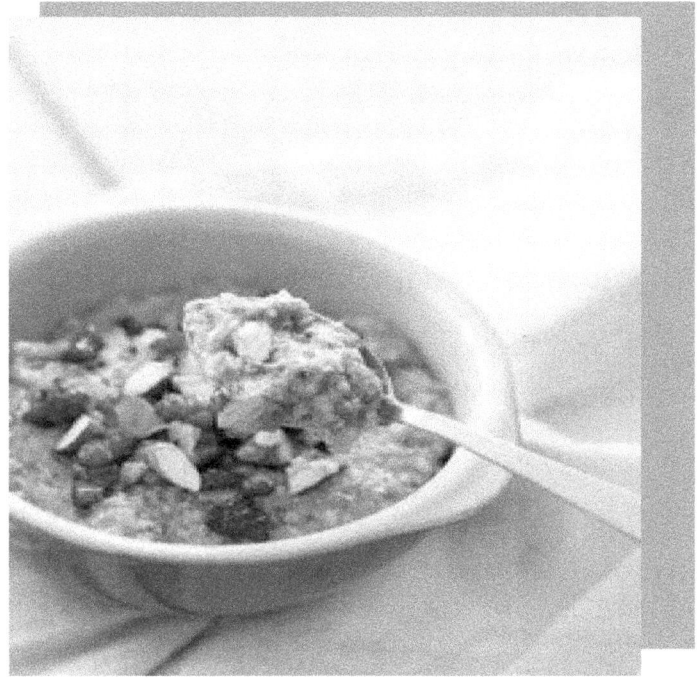

Preparation Time: 10 minutes
Servings: 1

Ingredients:
- ½ tsp vanilla extract

- ¼ tsp granulated stevia
- 1 tbsp chia seeds
- 1 tbsp flaxseed meal
- 2 tbsp unsweetened shredded coconut
- 2 tbsp almond flour
- 2 tbsp hemp hearts
- ½ cup water
- Pinch of salt

Directions:

1. Add all ingredients except vanilla extract to a saucepan and heat over low heat until thickened.
2. Stir well and serve warm.

Nutrition: Calories 370; Fat 30.2 g; Carbohydrates 12.8 g; Sugar 1.9 g; Protein 13.5 g; Cholesterol 0 mg;

Easy Chia Seed Pudding

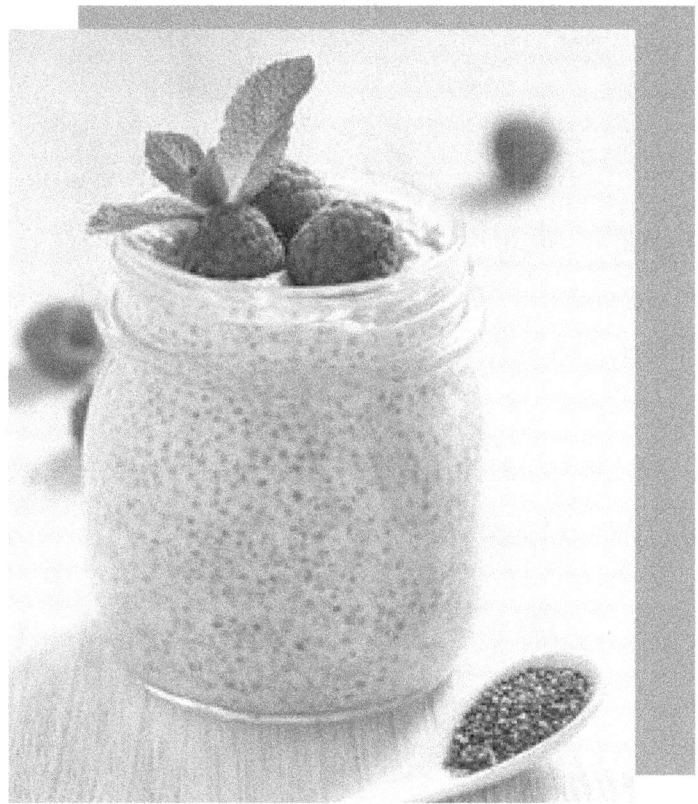

Preparation Time: 10 minutes

Servings: 4

Ingredients:
- ¼ tsp cinnamon
- 15 drops liquid stevia

- ½ tsp vanilla extract
- ½ cup chia seeds
- 2 cups unsweetened coconut milk

Directions:
1. Add all ingredients into the glass jar and mix well.
2. Close jar with lid and place in refrigerator for 4 hours.
3. Serve chilled and enjoy.

Nutrition: Calories 347; Fat 33.2 g; Carbohydrates 9.8 g; Sugar 4.1 g; Protein 5.9 g; Cholesterol 0 mg;

Cinnamon Noatmeal

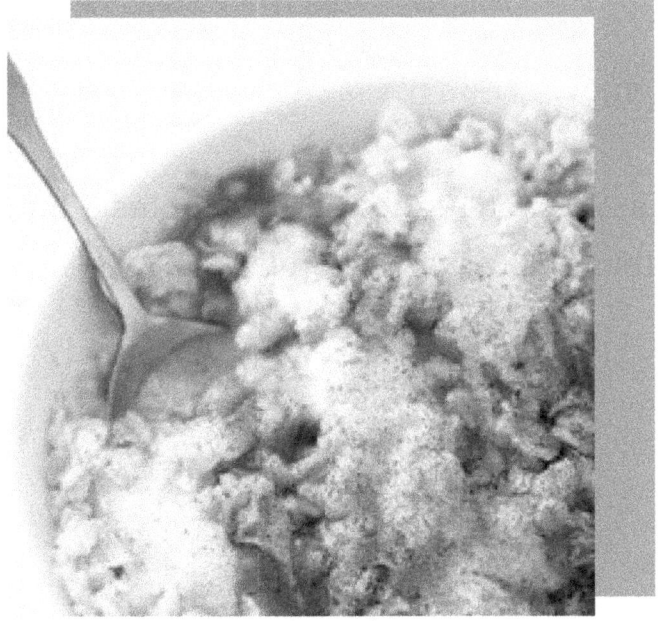

Preparation Time: 10 minutes

Servings: 2

Ingredients:
- ¾ cup hot water
- 2 tbsp sugar-free maple syrup
- ½ tsp ground cinnamon
- 2 tbsp ground flax seeds
- 3 tbsp vegan vanilla protein powder
- 3 tbsp hulled hemp seeds

Directions:
1. Add all ingredients into the bowl and stir until well combined.
2. Serve and enjoy.

Nutrition: Calories 220; Fat 12.5 g; Carbohydrates 9.5 g; Sugar 0.1 g; Protein 17.6 g; Cholesterol 0 mg;

Delicious Vegan Zoodles

Preparation Time: 15 minutes

Servings: 4

Ingredients:

- 4 small zucchinis, spiralized into noodles
- 3 tbsp vegetable stock
- 1 cup red pepper, diced
- 1/2 cup onion, diced
- 3/4 cup nutritional yeast
- 1 tbsp garlic powder
- Pepper
- Salt

Directions:

1. Add zucchini noodles, red pepper, and onion in a pan with vegetable stock and cook over medium heat for few minutes.
2. Add nutritional yeast and garlic powder and cook for few minutes until creamy.
3. Season with pepper and salt.
4. Stir well and serve.

Nutrition: Calories 71; Fat 0.9 g; Carbohydrates 12.1 g; Sugar 5.7 g; Protein 5.7 g; Cholesterol 0 mg;

Avocado Tofu Scramble

Preparation Time: 15 minutes

Servings: 1

Ingredients:
- 1 tbsp fresh parsley, chopped
- ½ medium avocado
- ½ block firm tofu, drained and crumbled
- ½ cup bell pepper, chopped
- ½ cup onion, chopped
- 1 tsp olive oil
- 1 tbsp water
- ¼ tsp cumin
- ¼ tsp garlic powder
- ¼ tsp paprika
- ¼ tsp turmeric
- 1 tbsp nutritional yeast
- Pepper
- Salt

Directions:
1. Heat olive oil to the pan over medium heat.
2. Add onion and bell pepper and sauté for 5 minutes.

3. Add crumbled tofu and nutritional yeast to the pan and sauté for 2 minutes.
4. Top with parsley and avocado.
5. Serve and enjoy.

Nutrition: Calories 164; Fat 9.7 g; Carbohydrates 15 g; Sugar 6 g; Protein 7.4 g; Cholesterol 0 mg;

Chia Raspberry Pudding Shots

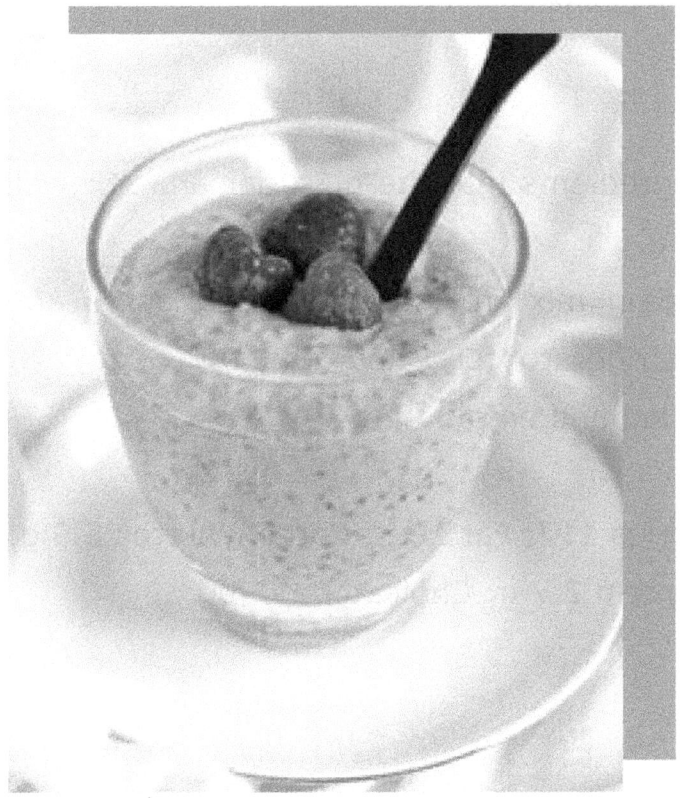

Preparation Time: 10 minutes

Servings: 4

Ingredients:

- ½ cup raspberries
- 10 drops liquid stevia
- 1 tbsp unsweetened cocoa powder

- ¼ cup unsweetened almond milk
- ½ cup unsweetened coconut milk
- ¼ cup chia seeds

Directions:
1. Add all ingredients into the glass jar and stir well to combine.
2. Pour pudding mixture into the shot glasses and place in refrigerator for 1 hour.
3. Serve chilled and enjoy.

Nutrition: Calories 117; Fat 10 g; Carbohydrates 5.9 g; Sugar 1.7 g; Protein 2.7 g; Cholesterol 0 mg;

Healthy Chia-Almond Pudding

Preparation Time: 10 minutes
Servings: 2

Ingredients:

- ½ tsp vanilla extract
- ¼ tsp almond extract
- 2 tbsp ground almonds
- 1 ½ cups unsweetened almond milk
- ¼ cup chia seeds

Directions:

1. Add chia seeds in almond milk and soak for 1 hour.
2. Add chia seed and almond milk into the blender.
3. Add remaining ingredients to the blender and blend until smooth and creamy.
4. Serve and enjoy.

Nutrition: Calories 138; Fat 10.2 g; Carbohydrates 6 g; Sugar 0.5 g; Protein 5.1 g; Cholesterol 0 mg;

Delicious Tofu Fries

Preparation Time: 50 minutes
Servings: 4

Ingredients:

- 15 oz firm tofu, drained, pressed and cut into long strips
- ¼ tsp garlic powder
- ¼ tsp onion powder
- ¼ tsp cayenne pepper
- ¼ tsp paprika
- ½ tsp oregano
- ½ tsp basil
- 2 tbsp olive oil
- Pepper
- Salt

Directions:
1. Preheat the oven to 190 C/ 375 F.
2. Add all ingredients into the large mixing bowl and toss well.
3. Place marinated tofu strips on a baking tray and

bake in preheated oven for 20 minutes.
4. Turn tofu strips to other side and bake for another 20 minutes.
5. Serve and enjoy.

Nutrition: Calories 137; Fat 11.5 g; Carbohydrates 2.3 g; Sugar 0.8 g; Protein 8.8 g; Cholesterol 0 mg;

Fresh Berries with Cream

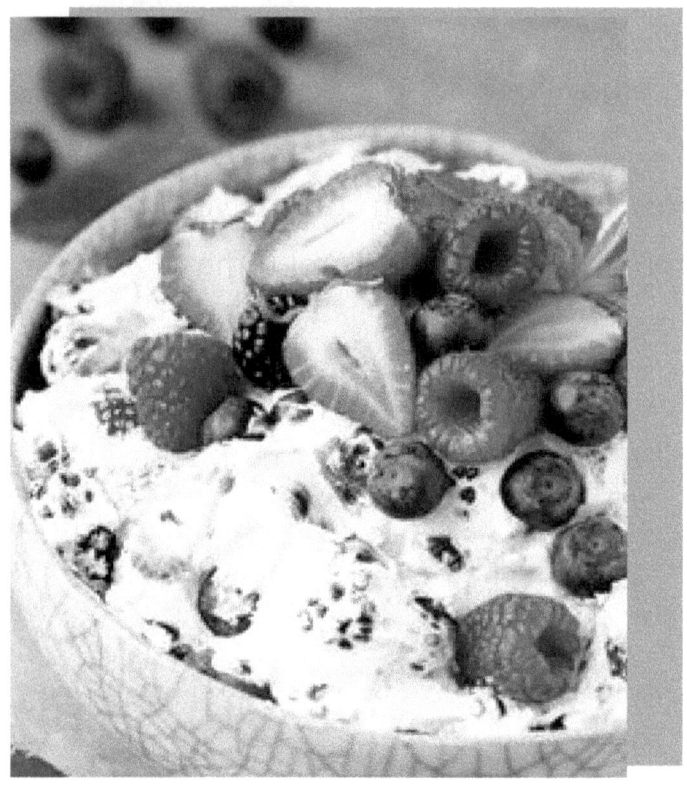

Preparation Time: 10 minutes

Servings: 1

Ingredients:

- 1/2 cup coconut cream
- 1 oz strawberries

- 1 oz raspberries
- 1/4 tsp vanilla extract

Directions:
1. Add all ingredients into the blender and blend until smooth.
2. Pour in serving bowl and top with fresh berries.
3. Serve and enjoy.

Nutrition: Calories 303; Fat 28.9 g; Carbohydrates 12 g; Sugar 6.8 g; Protein 3.3 g; Cholesterol 0 mg;

Almond Hemp Heart Porridge

Preparation Time: 10 minutes

Servings: 2

Ingredients:
- ¼ cup almond flour
- ½ tsp cinnamon
- ¾ tsp vanilla extract
- 5 drops stevia
- 1 tbsp chia seeds
- 2 tbsp ground flax seed
- ½ cup hemp hearts
- 1 cup unsweetened coconut milk

Directions:
1. Add all ingredients except almond flour to a saucepan. Stir to combine.
2. Heat over medium heat until just starts to lightly boil.
3. Once start bubbling then stir well and cook for 1 minute more.
4. Remove from heat and stir in almond flour.

5. Serve immediately and enjoy.

Nutrition: Calories 329; Fat 24.4 g; Carbohydrates 9.2 g; Sugar 1.8 g; Protein 16.2 g; Cholesterol 0 mg;

The Plant Based Lunch

Avocado & Radish Salad

Servings: 2

Preparation Time: 10 Minutes

Calories: 223

Protein: 3 Grams

Fat: 19 Grams

Carbs: 10 Grams

Ingredients:

- 1 Avocado, Sliced
- 6 Radishes, Sliced
- 2 Tomatoes, Sliced
- 1 Lettuce Head, Leaves Separated
- ½ Red Onion, Peeled & Sliced
-

Dressing:

- ½ Cup Olive Oil

- ¼ Cup Lime Juice, Fresh

- ¼ Cup Apple Cider Vinegar
- 3 Cloves Garlic, Chopped Fine
- Sea Salt & Black Pepper to Taste

Directions:

1. Spread your lettuce leaves on a platter, and then layer with your onion, tomatoes, avocado and radishes.
2. Whisk your dressing ingredients together before drizzling it over your salad.

Baked Okra & Tomato

Servings: 6

Preparation Time: 1 Hour 15 Minutes

Calories: 55

Protein: 3 Grams

Fat: 0 Grams

Carbs: 12 Grams

Ingredients:

- ½ cup Lime Beans, Frozen
- 4 Tomatoes, Chopped
- 8 Ounces Okra, Fresh, Washed & Stemmed, Sliced into ½ Inch Thick Slices
- 1 Onion, Sliced into Rings
- ½ Sweet Pepper, Seeded & Sliced Thin
- Pinch Crushed Red Pepper
- Sea Salt to taste
-

Directions:

1. Start by heating the oven to 350, and then cook your lime beans. Drain them, and then get out a

two-quarter casserole.
2. Combine everything together, and bake covered with foil for fort-five minutes.
3. Stir, and then uncover. Bake for another thirty minutes, and stir before serving.

Watercress & Blood Orange Salad

Servings: 4

Preparation Time: 10 Minutes

Calories: 94

Protein: 2 Grams

Fat: 5 Grams

Carbs: 13 Grams

Ingredients:

- 1 Tablespoon Hazelnuts, Toasted & Chopped
- 2 Blood Oranges (or Navel Oranges)
- 3 Cups watercress, Stems Removed
- 1/8 Teaspoon Sea Salt, Fine
- 1 Tablespoon Lemon Juice, Fresh
- 1 Tablespoon Honey, Raw
- 1 Tablespoon Water
- 2 Tablespoons Chives, Fresh

Directions:

1. Whisk your oil, honey, lemon juice, chives, salt and water together. Add in your watercress, tossing

until it's coated.
2. Arrange the mixture onto salad plates, and top with orange slices. Drizzle with remaining liquid, and sprinkle with hazelnuts.

Lentil Potato Salad

Servings: 2

Preparation Time: 35 Minutes

Calories: 400

Protein: 7 Grams

Fat: 26 Grams

Carbs: 39 Grams

Ingredients:

- ½ Cup Beluga Lentils
- 8 Fingerling Potatoes
- 1 Cup Scallions, Sliced Thin
- ¼ Cup Cherry Tomatoes, Halved
- ¼ Cup Lemon Vinaigrette
- Sea Salt & Black Pepper to Taste

Directions:

3. Bring two cups of water to simmer in a pot, adding your
4. lentils. Cook for twenty to twenty-five minutes, and then drain. Your lentils should be tender.

5. Bring another pot of salted water to a boil, and add in your potatoes. Reduce to a simmer, cooking for fifteen
6. minutes, and then drain. Halve your potatoes once they're cool enough to touch.
7. Put your lentils on a serving plate, and then top with scallions, potatoes and tomatoes. Drizzle with your vinaigrette, and season with salt and pepper.

Edamame Salad

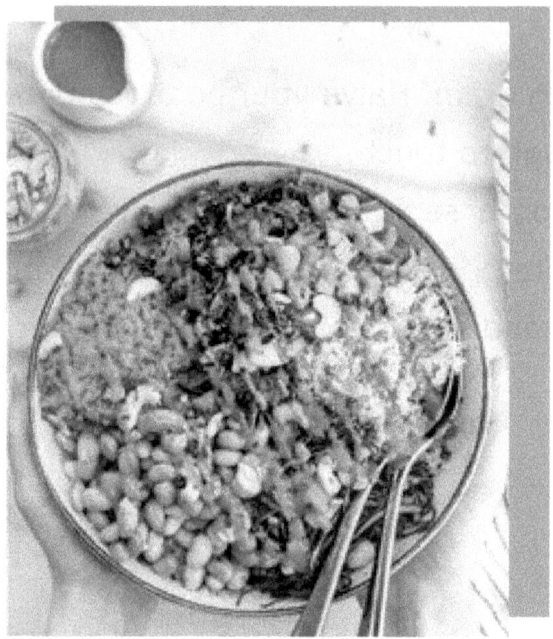

Servings: 1

Preparation Time: 15 Minutes

Calories: 299

Protein: 20 Grams

Fat: 9 Grams

Carbs: 38 Grams

Ingredients:

- ¼ Cup Red Onion, Chopped

- 1 Cup Corn Kernels, Fresh
- 1 Cup Edamame Beans, Shelled & Thawed
- 1 Red Bell Pepper, Chopped
- 2-3 Tablespoons Lime Juice, Fresh
- 5-6 Basil Leaves, Fresh & Sliced
- 5-6 Mint Leaves, Fresh & Sliced
- Sea Salt & Black Pepper to Taste

Directions:
1. Place everything into a Mason jar, and then seal the jar tightly.
2. Shake well before serving.

Cauliflower & Apple Salad

Servings: 4

Preparation Time: 25 Minutes

Calories: 198

Protein: 7 Grams

Fat: 8 Grams

Carbs: 32 Grams

Ingredients:

- 3 Cups Cauliflower, Chopped into Florets
- 2 Cups Baby Kale
- 1 Sweet Apple, Cored & Chopped
- ¼ Cup Basil, Fresh & Chopped
- ¼ Cup Mint, Fresh & Chopped
- ¼ Cup Parsley, Fresh & Chopped
- 1/3 Cup Scallions, Sliced Thin
- 2 Tablespoons Yellow Raisins
- 1 Tablespoon Sun Dried Tomatoes, Chopped
- ½ Cup Miso Dressing, Optional
- ¼ Cup Roasted Pumpkin Seeds, Optional

Directions:

Combine everything together, tossing before serving.

Olive & Fennel Salad

Servings: 3

Preparation Time: 5 Minutes

Calories: 331

Protein: 3 Grams

Fat: 29 Grams

Carbs: 15 Grams

Ingredients:

- 6 Tablespoons Olive Oil
- 3 Fennel Bulbs, Trimmed, Cored & Quartered
- 2 Tablespoons Parsley, Fresh & Chopped
- 1 Lemon, Juiced & Zested
- 12 Black Olives
- Sea Salt & Black Pepper to Taste

Directions:

1. Grease your baking dish, and then place your fennel in it. Make sure the cut side is up.
2. Mix your lemon zest, lemon juice, salt, pepper and oil, pouring it over your fennel.

3. Sprinkle your olives over it, and bake at 400.
4. Serve with parsley.

Red Pepper & Broccoli Salad

Servings: 2

Preparation Time: 15 Minutes

Calories: 185

Protein: 4 Grams

Fat: 14 Grams

Carbs: 8 Grams

Ingredients:

- Ounces Lettuce Salad Mix
- 1 Head Broccoli, Chopped into Florets
- 1 Red Pepper, Seeded & Chopped

Dressing:

- 3 Tablespoons White Wine Vinegar
- 1 Teaspoon Dijon Mustard
- 1 Clove Garlic, Peeled & Chopped Fine
- ½ Teaspoon Black Pepper
- ½ Teaspoon Sea Salt, Fine
- 2 Tablespoons Olive Oil
- 1 Tablespoon Parsley, Chopped

Directions:
1. Blanch your broccoli in boiling water, and then drain it. Drain it on a paper towel.
2. Whisk together all dressing ingredients.
3. Toss ingredients together before serving.

Zucchini & Lemon Salad

Servings: 2

Preparation Time: 3 Hours 10 Minutes

Calories: 159

Protein: 3 Grams

Fat: 14 Grams

Net Carbs: 7 Grams

Ingredients:

- 1 Green Zucchini, Sliced into Rounds
- 1 Yellow Squash, Zucchini, Sliced into Rounds
- 1 Clove Garlic, Peeled & Chopped
- 2 Tablespoons Olive Oil
- 2 Tablespoons Basil, Fresh
- 1 Lemon, Juiced & Zested
- ¼ Cup Coconut Milk
- Sea Salt & Black Pepper to Taste

Directions:

Toss all of your ingredients in a bowl, refrigerating for three hours before serving.

Mediterranean Wrap

Servings: 1

Preparation Time: 10 Minutes

Calories: 428

Protein: 13 Grams

Fat: 23 Grams

Carbs: 47 Grams

Ingredients:
- ¼ Cup Crispy Chickpeas
- ¼ Cup Cherry Tomatoes, Halved
- Handful Baby Spinach
- 2 Romaine Lettuce Leaves for Wrapping
- 2 Tablespoons Lemon Juice, Fresh
- ¼ Cup Hummus
- 2 Tablespoons Kalamata Olives, Quartered

Directions:
1. Mix everything but your lettuce leaves and hummus together.
2. Put your hummus on your lettuce leaves, topping

with your chickpea mixture, and then serve immediately.

Quinoa with Nectarine Slaw

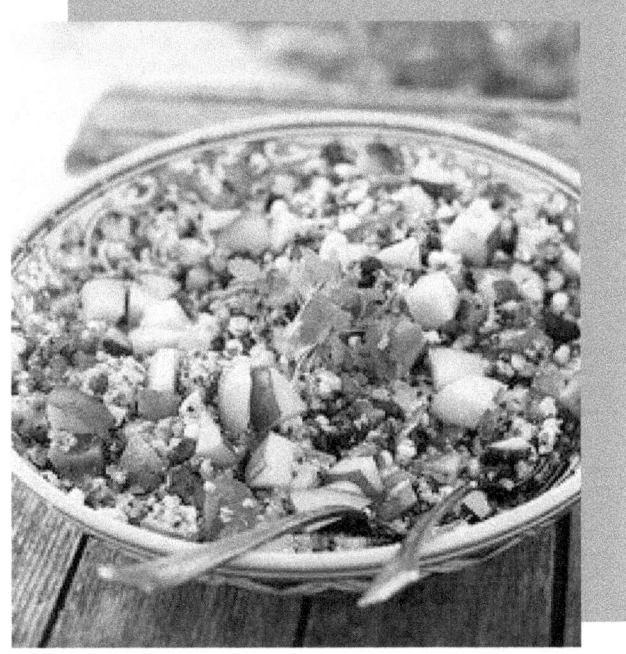

Servings: 2

Preparation Time: 20 Minutes

Calories: 396

Protein: 11 Grams

Fat: 18 Grams

Carbs: 52 Grams

Ingredients:

- ½ Cup Kale, Chopped
- 1/3 Cup Pumpkin Seeds, Roasted
- 3 Tablespoons Lemon Vinaigrette
- 1 Teaspoon Nutritional Yeast (Optional)
- 1/3 Cup Scallions, Sliced Thin
- 1 Cup Quinoa, Cooked & Room Temperature
- 2 Nectarines, Chopped into ½ Inch Wedges
- ½ Cup White Cabbage, Shredded

Directions:

Combine everything together in a bowl before serving.

Summer Chickpea Salad

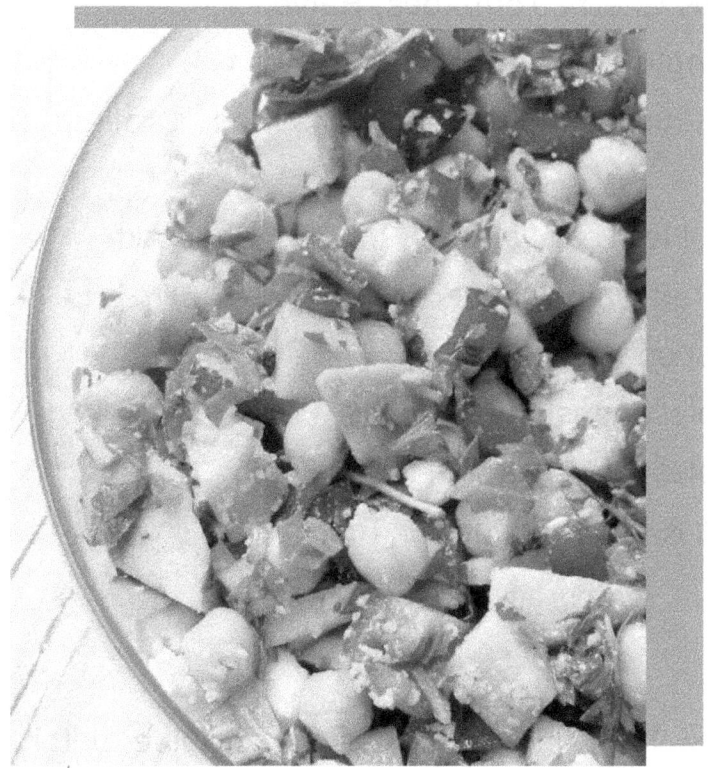

Servings: 4

Preparation Time: 15 Minutes

Calories: 145

Protein: 4 Grams

Fat: 7.5 Grams

Carbs: 16 Grams

Ingredients:

- 1 ½ Cups Cherry Tomatoes, Halved
- 1 Cup English Cucumber, Slices
- 1 Cup Chickpeas, Canned, Unsalted, Drained & Rinsed
- 1/3 Cup Flat Leaf Parsley, Roughly Chopped
- ¼ Cup Red Onion, Slivered
- 2 Tablespoon Olive Oil
- 1 ½ Tablespoons Lemon Juice, Fresh
- 1 ½ Tablespoons Lemon Juice, Fresh
- Sea Salt & Black Pepper to Taste

Directions:

Mix everything together, and toss to combine before serving.

Corn & Black Bean Salad

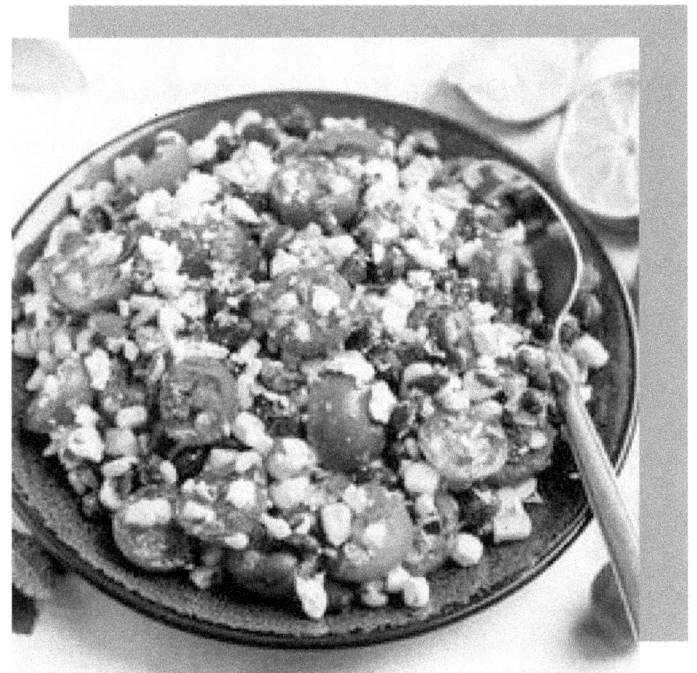

Servings: 6

Preparation Time: 10 Minutes

Calories: 159

Protein: 6.4 Grams

Fat: 5.6 Grams

Carbs: 23.7 Grams

Ingredients:

- ¼ Cup Cilantro, Fresh & Chopped
- 1 Can Corn, Drained (10 Ounces)
- 1/8 Cup Red Onion, Chopped
- 1 Can Black Beans, Drained (15 Ounces)
- 1 Tomato, Chopped
- 3 Tablespoons Lemon Juice, Fresh
- 2 Tablespoons Olive Oil
- Sea Salt & Black Pepper to Taste

Directions:

Mix everything together, and then refrigerate until cool. Serve cold.

Parsley Salad

Servings: 8

Preparation Time: 30 Minutes

Calories: 165.2

Protein: 3.8 Grams

Fat: 9.1 Grams

Carbs: 20.1 Grams

Ingredients:
- 3 Lemons, Juiced
- 150 Grams Flat Lea Parsley, Chopped Fine
- 1 Cup Boiled Water
- 5 Tablespoons Olive Oil
- Sea Salt & Black Pepper to Taste
- 6 Green Onions, Chopped Fine
- 1 Cup Bulgur
- 4 Tomatoes, Chopped Fine

Directions:
1. Add your Bulgur to your water, and mix well. Put a towel on top of it to steam it. Keep it to the side,

and then chop your spring onions, tomatoes and parsley. Put them in your salad bowl.
2. Pour your juice into the mixture, and then add in your olive oil, salt and pepper.
3. Put this mixture over your bulgur to serve.

Red Lentil Soup

Servings: 4

Preparation Time: 50 Minutes

Calories: 188

Protein: 12.5 Grams

Fat: 1.2 Grams

Carbs: 33.6 Grams

Ingredients:

- 1 Teaspoon Paprika
- 4 Cups Vegetable Stock
- ¼ Cup Onion, Chopped Fine
- 1 Cup Lentil, Red, Washed & Cleaned
- ½ Cup Potato, Peeled & Diced
- Sea Salt & Black Pepper to Taste

Directions:

1. Rinse your lentils under cold water, and then get out a medium pot.
2. Place your red lentils, potatoes, stock, onion and paprika in the pot.

3. Bring it to a boil, and then decrease the heat to allow it to simmer.
4. Put the lid on loosely, and cook until your lentils are tender. This will take roughly thirty minutes.
5. Add your salt and pepper, put a cup of the soup in the food processor, and then place the blended soup back into the pot.
6. Serve warm.

Dinner Recipes

Tofu & Asparagus Stir Fry

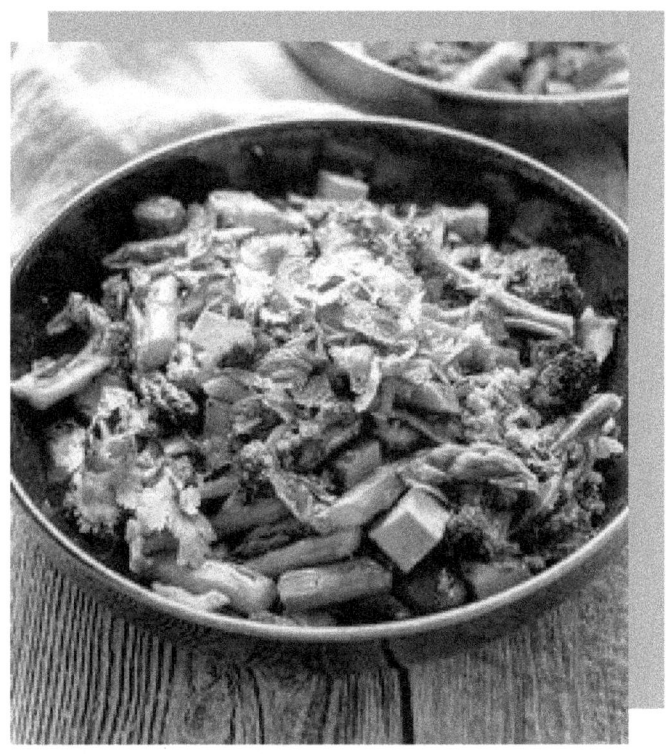

Servings: 3

Preparation Time: 20 Minutes

Calories: 380

Protein: 22 Grams

Fat: 24 Grams

Carbs: 27 Grams

Ingredients:

- 1 Tablespoon Ginger, Peeled & Grated
- 8 Ounces Firm Tofu, Chopped into Slices
- 4 Green Onions, Sliced Thin
- Toasted Sesame Oil to Taste
- 1 Bunch Asparagus, Trimmed & Chopped
- 1 Handful Cashew Nuts, Chopped & Toasted
- 2 Tablespoons Hoisin Sauce
- 1 Lime, Juiced & Zested
- 1 Handful Mint, Fresh & Chopped
- 1 Handful Basil, Fresh & Chopped
- 3 Cloves Garlic, Chopped
- 3 Handfuls Spinach, Chopped
- Pinch Sea Salt

Directions:

1. Get out a wok and heat up your oil. Add in your tofu, cooking for a few minutes.
2. Put your tofu to the side, and then sauté your red pepper flakes, ginger, salt, onions and asparagus for a minute.
3. Mix in your spinach, garlic, and cashews, cooking

for another two minutes.

4. Add your tofu back in, and then drizzle in your lime juice, lime zest, hoisin sauce, cooking for another half a minute.
5. Remove it from heat, adding in your mint and basil.

Cauliflower Steaks

Servings: 4

Preparation Time: 30 Minutes

Calories: 167

Protein: 6 Grams

Fat: 13 Grams

Carbs: 10 Grams

Ingredients:

- ¼ Teaspoon Black Pepper
- ½ Teaspoon Sea Salt, Fine
- 1 Tablespoon Olive Oil
- 1 Head Cauliflower, Large
- ¼ Cup Creamy Hummus
- 2 Tablespoons Lemon Sauce
- ½ Cup Peanuts, Crushed (Optional)
-

Directions:

1. Start by heating your oven to 425.
2. Cut your cauliflower stems, and then remove the leaves. Put the cut side down, and then slice half

down the middle. Cut into ¾ inch steaks. If you cut them thinner, they could fall apart.
3. Arrange them in a single layer on a baking sheet, drizzling with oil. Season with salt and pepper, and bake for twenty to twenty-five minutes. They should be lightly browned and tender.
4. Spread your hummus on the steaks, drizzling with your lemon sauce. Top with peanuts if you're using it.

Tofu Poke

Servings: 4

Preparation Time: 30 Minutes

Calories: 262

Protein: 16 Grams

Fat: 15 Grams

Carbs: 19 Grams

Ingredients:

- ¾ Cup Scallions, Sliced Thin
- 1 ½ Tablespoons Mirin
- ¼ Cup Tamari
- 1 ½ Tablespoon Dark Sesame Oil, Toasted
- 1 Tablespoon Sesame Seeds, Toasted (Optional)
- 2 Teaspoons Ginger, fresh & Grated
- ½ Teaspoon Red Pepper, crushed
- 12 Ounces Extra Firm Tofu, Drained & Cut into ½ Inch Pieces
- 4 Cups Zucchini Noodles
- 2 Tablespoons Rice Vinegar
- 2 Cups Carrots, Shredded
- 2 Cups Pea Shoots

- ¼ Cup Basil, Fresh & Chopped
- ¼ Cup Peanuts, Toasted & Chopped (Optional)

Directions:

1. Wisk your tamari, mirin, sesame seeds, oil, ginger, red pepper, and scallion greens in a bowl. Set two tablespoons of this sauce aside, and add the tofu to the remaining sauce. Toss to coat.
2. Combine your vinegar and zucchini noodles in a bowl.
3. Divide it between four bowls, topping with tofu, carrots, and a tablespoon of basil and peanuts.
4. Drizzle with sauce before serving.

Ratatouille

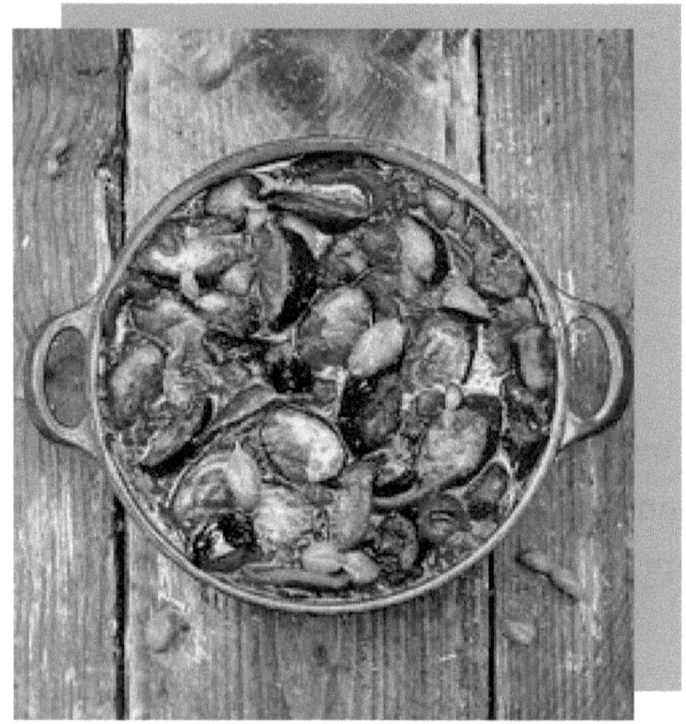

Servings: 10

Preparation Time: 1 Hour 15 Minutes

Calories: 90
Protein: 3 Grams
Fat: 25 Grams
Carbs: 13 Grams

Ingredients:

- 2 Tablespoons Olive Oil
- 2 Eggplants, Peeled & Cubed
- 8 Zucchini, Chopped
- 4 Tomatoes, Chopped
- ¼ Cup Basil, Chopped
- 4 Thyme Sprigs
- 2 Yellow Onions, Diced
- 3 Cloves Garlic, Minced
- 3 Bell Peppers, Chopped
- 1 Bay Leaf
- Sea Salt to Taste

Directions:

1. Salt your eggplant and leave it in a strainer.
2. Heat a teaspoon of oil in a Dutch oven, cooking your onions for ten minutes. Season with salt.
3. Mix your peppers in, cooking for five more minutes.
4. Place this mixture in a bowl.
5. Heat your oil and sauté zucchini, sprinkling with salt. Cook for five minutes, and place it in the same bowl.
6. Rinse your eggplant, squeezing the water out, and

heat another two teaspoons of oil in your Dutch oven. Cook your eggplant for ten minutes, placing it in your vegetable bowl.
7. Heat the remaining oil and cook your garlic. Add in your tomatoes, thyme sprigs and bay leaves to deglaze the bottom.
8. Toss your vegetables back in, and then bring it to a simmer.
9. Simmer for forty-five minutes, and make sure to stir. Discard your thyme and bay leaf. Mix in your basil and serve warm.

Tomato Gazpacho

Servings: 6

Preparation Time: 2 Hours 25 Minutes

Calories: 181
Protein: 3 Grams
Fat: 14 Grams
Carbs: 14 Grams

Ingredients:

- 2 Tablespoons + 1 Teaspoon Red Wine Vinegar, Divided
- ½ Teaspoon Pepper
- 1 Teaspoon Sea Salt
- 1 Avocado,
- ¼ Cup Basil, Fresh & Chopped
- 3 Tablespoons + 2 Teaspoons Olive Oil, Divided
- 1 Clove Garlic, crushed
- 1 Red Bell Pepper, Sliced & Seeded
- 1 Cucumber, Chunked
- 2 ½ lbs. Large Tomatoes, Cored & Chopped

Directions:

1. Place half of your cucumber, bell pepper, and ¼ cup of each tomatoes in a bowl, covering. Set it in the fried.
2. Puree your remaining tomatoes, cucumber and bell pepper with garlic, three tablespoons oil, two tablespoons of vinegar, sea salt and black pepper into a blender, blending until smooth. Transfer it to a bowl, and chill for two hours.
3. Chop the avocado, adding it to your chopped vegetables, adding your remaining oil, vinegar, salt, pepper and basil.
4. Ladle your tomato puree mixture into bowls, and serve with chopped vegetables as a salad.

Simple Chili

Servings: 4

Preparation Time: 30 Minutes

Calories: 160

Protein: 8 Grams

Fat: 3 Grams

Carbs: 29 Grams

Ingredients:
- 1 Onion, Diced
- 1 Teaspoon Olive Oil
- 3 Cloves Garlic, Minced
- 28 Ounces Tomatoes, Canned
- ¼ Cup Tomato Paste
- 14 Ounces Kidney Beans, Canned, Rinsed & Dried
- 2-3 Teaspoons Chili Powder
- ¼ Cup Cilantro, Fresh (or Parsley)
- ¼ Teaspoon Sea Salt, Fine

Directions:
1. Get out a pot, and sauté your onion and garlic in

your oil

2. at the bottom cook for five minutes. Add in your tomato paste, tomatoes, beans, and chili powder. Season with salt.
3. Allow it to simmer for ten to twenty minutes.
4. Garnish with cilantro or parsley to serve.

Cauliflower Rice Tabbouleh

Servings: 4

Preparation Time: 20 Minutes

Calories: 220

Protein: 7 Grams

Fat: 15 Grams

Carbs: 20 Grams

Ingredients:

- 4 Cups Cauliflower Rice
- 1 ½ Cups Cherry Tomatoes, Quartered
- 3-4 Tablespoons Olive Oil
- 1 Cup Parsley, Fresh & Chopped
- 1 Cup Mint, Fresh & Chopped
- 1 Cup Snap Peas, Sliced Thin
- 1 Small Cucumber, Cut into ¼ Inch Pieces
- ¼ Cup Scallions, Sliced Thin
- 3-4 Tablespoons Lemon Juice, Fresh
- 1 Teaspoon Sea Salt, Fine
- ½ Teaspoon Black Pepper

Directions:

1. Get out a bowl and combine your cauliflower rice, tomatoes, mint, parsley, cucumbers, scallions and snap peas together. Toss until combined.
2. Add your olive oil and lemon juice before tossing again. Season with salt and pepper.

Dijon Maple Burgers

Servings: 12

Preparation Time: 50 Minutes

Calories: 200

Protein: 8 Grams

Fat: 11 Grams

Carbs: 21 Grams

Ingredients:

- 1 Red Bell Pepper
- 19 Ounces Can Chickpeas, Rinsed & Drained
- 1 Cup Almonds, Ground
- 2 Teaspoons Dijon Mustard
- 1 Teaspoon Oregano
- ½ Teaspoon Sage
- 1 Cup Spinach, Fresh
- 1 – ½ Cups Rolled Oats
- 1 Clove Garlic, Pressed
- ½ Lemon, Juiced
- 2 Teaspoons Maple Syrup, Pure
-

Directions:

1. Start by heating your oven to 350, and then get out a baking sheet. Line it with parchment paper.
2. Cut your red pepper in half and then take the seeds out. Place it on your baking sheet, and roast in the oven while you prepare your other ingredients.
3. Process your chickpeas, almonds, mustard and maple syrup together in a food processor.
4. Add in your lemon juice, oregano, sage, garlic and spinach, processing again. Make sure it's combined, but don't puree it.
5. Once your red bell pepper is softened, which should roughly take ten minutes, add this to the processor as well. Add in your oats, mixing well.
6. Form twelve patties, cooking in the oven for a half hour. They should be browned.

Sushi Bowl

Servings: 1

Preparation Time: 40 Minutes

Calories: 467

Protein: 22 Grams

Fat: 20 Grams

Carbs: 56 Grams

Ingredients:

- ½ Cup Edamame Beans, Shelled & Fresh
- ¾ Cup Brown Rice, Cooked
- ½ Cup Spinach, Chopped
- ¼ Cup Bell Pepper, Sliced
- ¼ Cup Avocado, Sliced
- ¼ Cup Cilantro, Fresh & Chopped
- 1 Scallion, Chopped
- ¼ Nori Sheet
- 1-2 Tablespoons Tamari
- 1 Tablespoon Sesame Seeds, Optional

Directions:

1. Steam your edamame beans, and then assemble your edamame, rice, avocado, spinach, cilantro, scallions and bell pepper into a bowl.
2. Cut the nori into ribbons, sprinkling it on top, drizzling with tamari and sesame seeds before serving.

Pesto & Tomato Quinoa

Servings: 1

Preparation Time: 25 Minutes

Calories: 535

Protein: 20 Grams

Fat: 23 Grams

Carbs: 69 Grams

Ingredients:

- 1 Teaspoon Olive Oil
- 1 Cup Onion, Chopped
- 1 Cup Zucchini, Chopped
- 1 Clove Garlic, Minced
- 1 Tomato, Chopped
- Pinch Sea Salt
- 2 Tablespoons Sun Dried Tomatoes, Chopped
- 2-3 Tablespoons Basil Pesto
- 1 Cup Spinach, Chopped
- 2 Cups Quinoa, Cooked
- 1 Tablespoon Nutritional Yeast, Optional

Directions:

1. Heat your oil in a skillet, and sauté your onion over medium-high heat. This should take five minutes, and then add in your garlic, cooking for another minute. Add in your sea salt and zucchini.
2. Cook for about five-minute and then add in your sun-dried tomatoes, and mix well.
3. Toss your pesto in, and then mix well.
4. Layer your spinach, quinoa and then zucchini mixture on a plate, topping with nutritional yeast if desired.

Sesame Bok Choy

Servings: 4

Preparation Time: 13 Minutes

Calories: 76

Protein: 4.4 Grams

Fat: 2.7 Grams

Carbs: 9.8 Grams

Ingredients:

- 1 Head Bok Choy
- 1 Teaspoon Canola Oil
- 1/3 Cup Green Onion, Chopped
- 1 Tablespoon Brown Sugar
- 1 ½ Tablespoon Soy Sauce, Light
- 1 Tablespoon Rice Wine
- ½ Teaspoon Ginger, Ground
- 1 Tablespoon Sesame Seeds

Directions:

1. Cut the stems and tops of your bok choy into one inch pieces.

2. Mix together all remaining ingredients in a bowl.
3. Add your bok choy, and top with your dressing.
4. Fry until tender, which should take eight to ten minutes.

Stuffed Bell Pepper

Servings: 4

Preparation Time: 25 Minutes

Calories: 126

Protein: 3 Grams

Fat: 5 Grams

Carbs: 19 Grams

Ingredients:

- 4 Bell Peppers, Halved & Hollowed
- ½ Cup Quinoa, Cooked
- 12 Black Olives, Halved
- 1/3 Cup Tomatoes, Sun Dried
- ½ Cup Baby Spinach
- 2 Cloves Garlic, Minced
- Sea Salt & Black Pepper to Taste

Directions:

1. Bake your peppers at 400 for ten minutes, and then mix the rest of your ingredients in a bowl.
2. Stuff your peppers with the quinoa mixture.

Cabbage & Beet Stew

Servings: 4

Preparation Time: 30 Minutes

Calories: 95

Protein: 1 Gram

Fat: 7 Grams

Carbs: 10 Grams

Ingredients:

- 2 Tablespoons Olive Oil
- 3 Cups Vegetable Broth
- 2 Tablespoons Lemon Juice, Fresh
- ½ Teaspoon Garlic Powder
- ½ Cup Carrots, Shredded
- 2 Cups Cabbage, Shredded
- 1 Cup Beets, Shredded
- Dill for Garnish
- ½ Teaspoon Onion Powder
- Sea Salt & Black Pepper to Taste

Directions:

1. Start by heating up your oil in a pot, and then sauté your vegetables.
2. Pour your broth in, mixing in your seasoning. Simmer until it's cooked through, and then top with dill.

Black Bean Burgers

Servings: 6

Preparation Time: 25 Minutes

Calories: 173

Protein: 7.3 Grams

Fat: 3.2 Grams

Carbs: 29.7 Grams

Ingredients:

- 1 Onion, Diced
- ½ Cup Corn Nibs
- 2 Cloves Garlic, Minced
- ½ Teaspoon Oregano, Dried
- ½ Cup Flour
- 1 Jalapeno Pepper, Small
- 2 Cups Black Beans, Mashed & Canned
- ¼ Cup Breadcrumbs (Vegan)
- 2 Teaspoons Parsley, Minced
- ¼ Teaspoon Cumin
- 1 Tablespoon Olive Oil
- 2 Teaspoons Chili Powder
- ½ Red Pepper, Diced

- Sea Salt to Taste

Directions:
1. Set your flour on a plate, and then get out your garlic, onion, peppers and oregano, throwing it in a pan. Cook over medium-high heat, and then cook until the onions are translucent. Place the peppers in, and sauté until tender.
2. Cook for two minutes, and then set it to the side.
3. Use a potato masher to mash your black beans, and then stir in the vegetables, cumin, breadcrumbs, parsley, salt and chili powder, and then divide it into six patties.
4. Coat each side, and then cook until it's fried on each side. It should take ten minutes. It should be cooked all the way through.

Grilled Eggplant Steaks

Servings: 6

Preparation Time: 35 Minutes

Calories: 86

Protein: 8 Grams

Fat: 7 Grams

Carbs: 12 Grams

Ingredients:

- 4 Roma Tomatoes, Diced
- 8 Ounces Feta, Diced
- 2 Eggplants
- 1 Tablespoon Olive Oil
- 1 Cup Parsley, Chopped
- 1 Cucumber, Diced
- Sea Salt & Black Pepper to Taste

Directions:

1. Slice your eggplants into three thick steaks, and then drizzle with oil. Season it with salt and pepper, and then grill for four minutes per side in a pan.

2. Top with the remaining ingredients.

Vegetable Stir Fry

Servings: 10

Preparation Time: 25 Minutes

Calories: 50

Protein: 2 Grams

Fat: 2 Grams

Carbs: 6 Grams

Ingredients:

- 1 Tablespoon Oil
- 1 Onion, Sliced
- 1 Cup Carrots, Sliced
- 2 Cups Sugar Snap Peas
- 2 Cups Broccoli Florets
- 1 Bell Pepper, Cut into Strips
- 1 Tablespoon Soy Sauce
- 1 Teaspoon Garlic, Minced

Directions:

1. Combine your carrots and onion into your wok, adding in your oil. Stir fry for two minutes, and

then add in the rest of your vegetables.
2. Stir for another seven minutes, and then add in your garlic and soy sauce. Stir fry until blended and hot.

Fried Pineapple Rice

Servings: 6

Preparation Time: 30 Minutes

Calories: 179

Protein: 3 Grams

Fat: 4.4 Grams

Carbs: 32.6 Grams

Ingredients:

- 2-3 Cups Brown Rice, Cooked & Cooled
- 1 Tablespoon Sesame Oil
- 2 Tablespoons Raisins (Optional)
- 1 Onion, Small & Chopped
- ½ -3/4 Cup Pineapple, Chopped
- 1 Tablespoon Soy Sauce (Or Braggs Liquid Amino)
- ½ Teaspoon Turmeric
- 1 Tomato, Chopped
- 1 Teaspoon Curry Powder
- 2 Tablespoons Cilantro, Fresh & Chopped
- Sea Salt & Black Pepper to Taste

Directions:

1. Start by getting out a sauce pan, and then add your sesame oil to the pan. Sauté your onions until they turn translucent.
2. Add in your cooked rice, soy sauce, pineapple, curry powder and turmeric.
3. Mix well and cook for eight to ten minutes.
4. Serve with cilantro, and season with salt and pepper.

Soup Salads And Sides

Cauliflower Coconut Rice

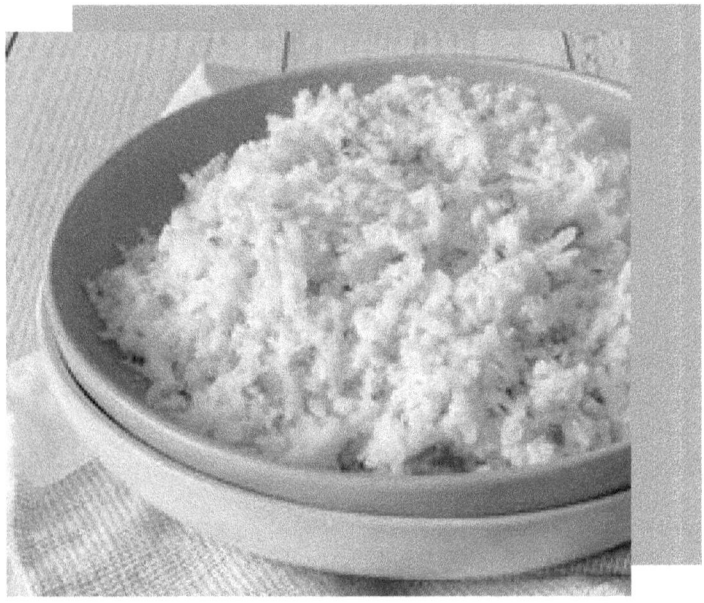

Preparation Time: 20 minutes

Servings: 3

Ingredients:

- 3 cups cauliflower rice
- ½ tsp onion powder
- 1 tsp chili paste

- 2/3 cup coconut milk
- Salt

Directions:
1. Add all ingredients to the pan and heat over medium-low heat. Stir to combine.
2. Cook for 10 minutes. Stir after every 2 minutes.
3. Remove lid and cook until excess liquid absorbed.
4. Serve and enjoy.

Nutrition: Calories 155; Fat 13.1 g; Carbohydrates 9.2 g; Sugar 4.8 g; Protein 3.4 g; Cholesterol 1 mg;

Fried Okra

Preparation Time: 20 minutes

Servings: 4

Ingredients:

- 1 lb. fresh okra, cut into ¼" slices
- 1/3 cup almond meal
- Pepper
- Salt
- Oil for frying

Directions:

1. Heat oil in large pan over medium-high heat.
2. In a bowl, mix together sliced okra, almond meal, pepper, and salt until well coated.
3. Once the oil is hot then add okra to the hot oil and cook until lightly browned.
4. Remove fried okra from pan and allow to drain on paper towels.
5. Serve and enjoy.

Nutrition: Calories 91; Fat 4.2 g; Carbohydrates 10.2 g; Sugar 10.2 g; Protein 3.9 g; Cholesterol 0 mg;

Asparagus Mash

Preparation Time: 20 minutes

Servings: 2

Ingredients:

- 10 asparagus shoots, chopped
- 1 tsp lemon juice
- 2 tbsp fresh parsley
- 2 tbsp coconut cream
- 1 small onion, diced
- 1 tbsp coconut oil
- Pepper
- Salt

Directions:

1. Sauté onion in coconut oil until onion is softened.
2. Blanch chopped asparagus in hot water for 2 minutes and drain immediately.
3. Add sautéed onion, lemon juice, parsley, coconut cream, asparagus, pepper, and salt into the blender and blend until smooth.
4. Serve warm and enjoy.

Nutrition: Calories 125; Fat 10.6 g; Carbohydrates 7.5 g; Sugar 3.6 g; Protein 2.6 g; Cholesterol 0 mg;

Baked Asparagus

Preparation Time: 25 minutes

Servings: 4

Ingredients:

- 40 asparagus spears
- 2 tbsp vegetable seasoning
- 2 tbsp garlic powder
- 2 tbsp salt

Directions:

1. Preheat the oven to 450 F/ 232 C.
2. Arrange all asparagus spears on baking tray and season with vegetable seasoning, garlic powder, and salt.
3. Place in preheated oven and bake for 20 minutes.
4. Serve warm and enjoy.

Nutrition: Calories 75; Fat 0.9 g; Carbohydrates 13.5 g; Sugar 5.5 g; Protein 6.7 g; Cholesterol 0 mg;

Spinach with Coconut Milk

Preparation Time: 25 minutes

Servings: 6

Ingredients:

- 16 oz spinach
- 2 tsp curry powder
- 13.5 oz coconut milk
- 1 tsp lemon zest
- ½ tsp salt

Directions:

1. Add spinach in pan and heat over medium heat. Once it is hot then add curry paste and few tablespoons of coconut milk. Stir well.
2. Add remaining coconut milk, lemon zest, and salt and cook until thickened.
3. Serve and enjoy.

Nutrition: Calories 167; Fat 15.6 g; Carbohydrates 6.7 g; Sugar 2.5 g; Protein 3.7 g; Cholesterol 0 mg;

Delicious Cabbage Steaks

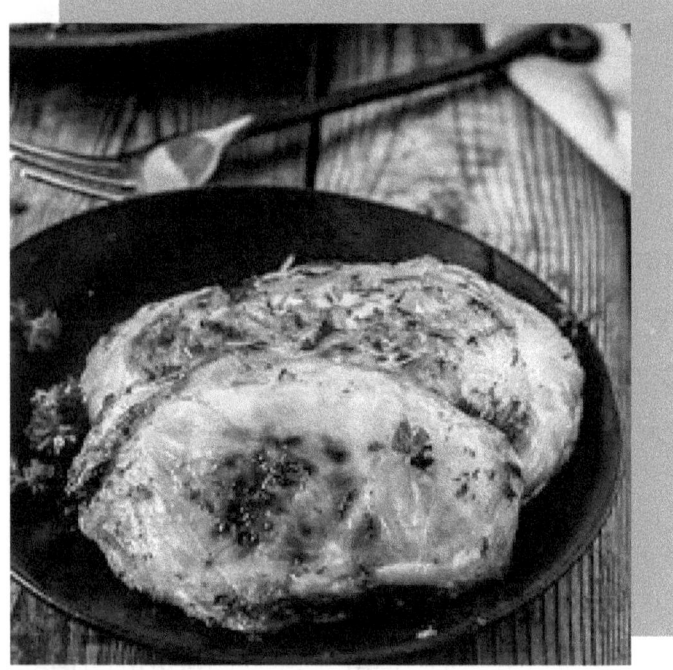

Preparation Time: 1 hour 10 minutes

Servings: 6

Ingredients:

- 1 medium cabbage head, slice 1" thick
- 2 tbsp olive oil
- 1 tbsp garlic, minced
- Pepper
- Salt

Directions:
1. In a small bowl, mix together garlic and olive oil.
2. Brush garlic and olive oil mixture onto both sides of sliced cabbage.
3. Season cabbage slices with pepper and salt.
4. Place cabbage slices onto a baking tray and bake at 350 F/ 180 C for 1 hour. Turn after 30 minutes.
5. Serve and enjoy.

Nutrition: Calories 72; Fat 4.8 g; Carbohydrates 7.4 g; Sugar 3.8 g; Protein 1.6 g; Cholesterol 0 mg;

Garlic Zucchini Squash

Preparation Time: 20 minutes

Servings: 4

Ingredients:
- 1 small squash, sliced
- 2 tbsp fresh basil, chopped
- 2 tbsp olive oil
- 1 garlic clove, chopped
- 1 large onion, sliced
- 2 fresh tomatoes, cut into wedges
- 1 small zucchini, sliced
- Pepper
- Salt

Directions:
1. Heat olive oil in a pan over medium-high heat.
2. Add onion, squash, zucchini, and garlic and sauté until lightly brown.
3. Add basil and tomatoes and cook for 5 minutes. Season with pepper and salt.
4. Simmer over low heat until squash is tender.
5. Stir well and serve.

Nutrition: Calories 97; Fat 7.2 g; Carbohydrates 8.2 g; Sugar 4.4 g; Protein 1.4 g; Cholesterol 0 mg;

Tomato Avocado Cucumber Salad

Preparation Time: 10 minutes

Servings: 4

Ingredients:
- 1 cucumber, sliced
- 2 avocado, chopped
- ½ onion, sliced
- 2 tomatoes, chopped
- 1 bell pepper, chopped
- For dressing:
- 2 tbsp cilantro
- ¼ tsp garlic powder
- 2 tbsp olive oil
- 1 tbsp lemon juice
- ½ tsp black pepper
- ½ tsp salt

Directions:
1. In a small bowl, mix together all dressing ingredients and set aside.
2. Add all salad ingredients into the large mixing bowl and mix well.

3. Pour dressing over salad and toss well.
4. Serve immediately and enjoy.

Nutrition: Calories 130; Fat 9.8 g; Carbohydrates 10.6 g; Sugar 5.1 g; Protein 2.1 g; Cholesterol 0 mg;

Cabbage Coconut Salad

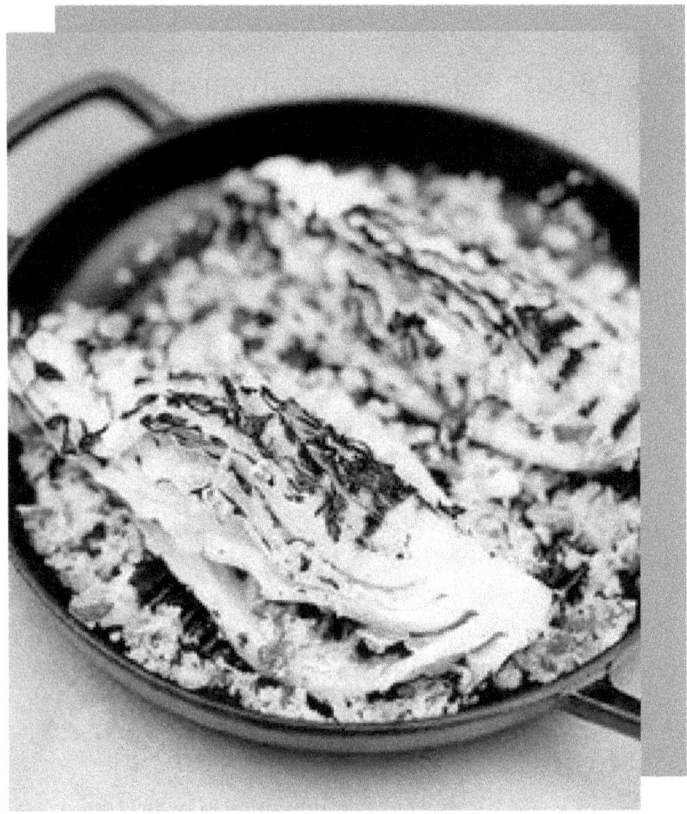

Preparation Time: 15 minutes

Servings: 4

Ingredients:
- 1/3 cup unsweetened desiccated coconut
- ½ medium head cabbage, shredded
- 2 tsp sesame seeds

- ¼ cup tamari sauce
- ¼ cup olive oil
- 1 fresh lemon juice
- ½ tsp cumin
- ½ tsp curry powder
- ½ tsp ginger powder

Directions:
1. Add all ingredients into the large mixing bowl and toss well.
2. Place salad bowl in refrigerator for 1 hour.
3. Serve and enjoy.

Nutrition: Calories 197; Fat 16.6 g; Carbohydrates 11.4 g; Sugar 7.1 g; Protein 3.5 g; Cholesterol 0 mg;

Asian Cucumber Salad

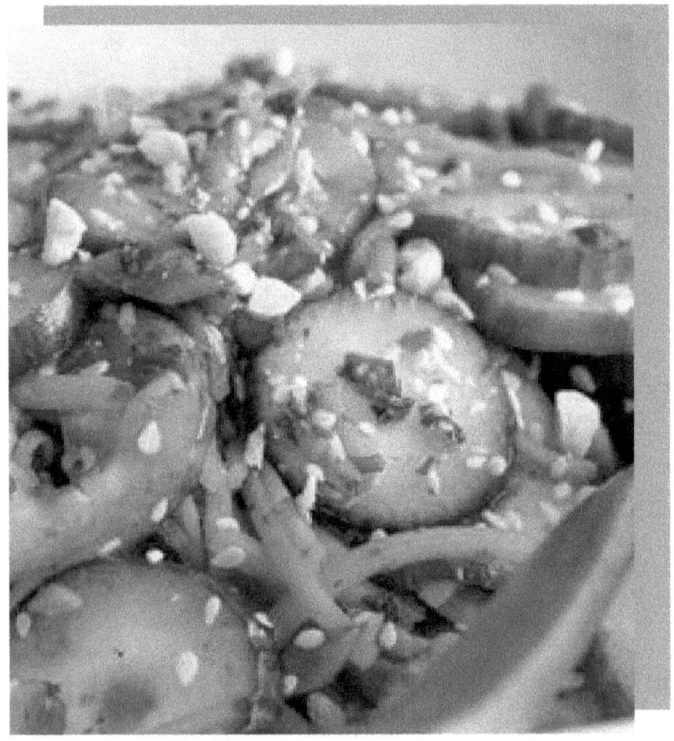

Preparation Time: 10 minutes

Servings: 6

Ingredients:

- 4 cups cucumbers, sliced
- ¼ tsp red pepper flakes
- ½ tsp sesame oil
- 1 tsp sesame seeds

- ¼ cup rice wine vinegar
- ¼ cup red pepper, diced
- ¼ cup onion, sliced
- ½ tsp sea salt

Directions:

Add all ingredients into the mixing bowl and toss well. Serve immediately and enjoy.

Nutrition: Calories 27; Fat 0.7 g; Carbohydrates 3.5 g; Sugar 1.6 g; Protein 0.7 g; Cholesterol 0 mg;

www.ingramcontent.com/pod-product-compliance
Lightning Source LLC
Chambersburg PA
CBHW071112030426
42336CB00013BA/2048